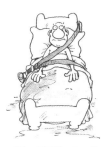

The Little Book
of Loony Sex Laws

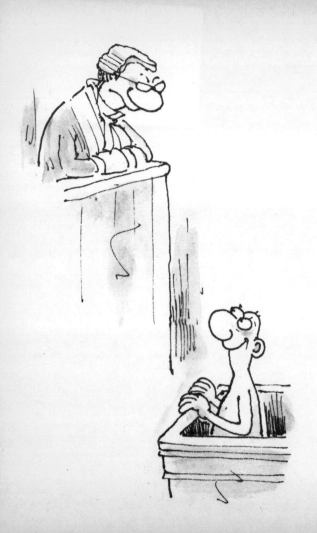

The Little Book of Loony Sex Laws

Christine Green

illustrated by

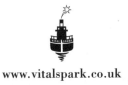

www.vitalspark.co.uk

The Vital Spark is an imprint of
Neil Wilson Publishing Ltd
303 The Pentagon Centre
36 Washington Street
GLASGOW
G3 8AZ

Tel: 0141-221-1117
Fax: 0141-221-5363
E-mail: info@nwp.co.uk
www.nwp.co.uk

A catalogue record for this book is
available from the British Library.

ISBN 1-903238-73-0

Typeset in Bodoni
Designed by Mark Blackadder

Printed in Poland

Contents

Loony Sex Laws

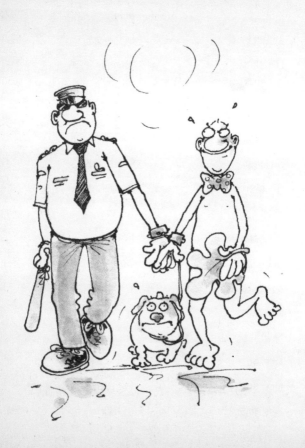

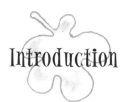

Introduction

SEX ... our most basic need and the driving force that has defined the evolution of all living things on this planet for millennia. Is it any surprise then that man has sought to try and control our sexual behaviour and, in doing so, has simply created a vast amount of largely unenforceable legislation? We all understand and approve of any laws created to protect infants and minors from the approaches of unsuitable and unsavoury characters, but why on earth pass a law that prohibits sexual intercourse while riding a motorcycle! That's clearly why you never see this happening in London, England!

Of the 34 countries surveyed in 2003 by a leading condom company, the top three places for sexual activity went to Hungary, Bulgaria and Russia. The Hungarians managed to have sex a staggering 152 times a year! The passionate French were fifth but could only be bothered 144 times a year and the Brits lagged graciously in 11th position. Canada shared joint 23rd with Italy and the USA lay at 25th with a measly 118 times a year on the bonkometer!

Perhaps the huge number of 'thou shalt not' sex laws on the statute books in the USA explains their poor performance. But what is extraordinary is the way that religion deals with sex. We all know what the Pope's position on contraception and abortion is, and we all know how dreadfully guilty young catholic boys become when they're passing through puberty into adulthood and confessing all sorts of secretory secrets to their priests. But did you know that for every awkward sexual situation, the Moslems have an answer? What is apparent from this compilation of loony sex laws is that the more loony they are, the less likely they are to work. But don't take my word for it, take a dip into the truly loony world of sex laws!

Christine Green

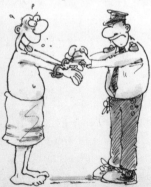

In Afghanistan...

... a rather unusual law sanctioned by the
Taliban militia banned all females from wearing
white socks which was supposed to deter men
from being physically attracted to them.

In Australia...

... an old law found in Melbourne's legal
archives related to men with a fetish for wearing
women's dresses. But not all dresses ... only
strapless ones! Lawmakers saw no problem in
allowing cross-dressing so long as the dresses
had sleeves.

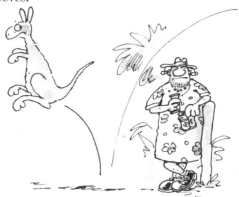

Loony Sex Laws

In Bahrain...

... should a male doctor need to examine a female's genitalia for medical reasons, he cannot look at them directly. Under the law he can only conduct the examination using a mirror in order to see the reflection.

In Bhutan...

... it was illegal for a younger brother to lose his virginity before his older brother. Furthermore the younger brother could not take a bride before his older sibling.

In Bolivia...

... in Santa Cruz a prostitute cannot solicit potential clients on the streets or in other public areas.

In Canada...

... in Winnipeg nudity within one's own home is banned unless all blinds and curtains are drawn.

Loony Sex Laws

In China...

... there are no laws against prostitution. According to a member of the Foreign Ministry in Beijing, 'There is no prostitution in China. However, we do have some women who make love for money.'

... women are prohibited from walking around a hotel room naked. The only place where she may be unclad is in the privacy of her bathroom.

... in Beijing it is illegal for a foreigner to take a Chinese woman to his hotel room for sex.

In Colombia...

... it is legal in Cali for a daughter's mother to be present in the same room on her first night of wedlock.

... there is a lot of old legislation that relates to the acts of adultery, some of which are still enforced. For instance, if a husband finds his wife in bed with a lover he is well within his rights to murder his wife because this is regarded as an *excusable act of passion*.

... it is not safe for any young woman to be alone on the streets in Bogota after sunset because it might be assumed that they are prostitutes and be subject to immediate arrest.

In Costa Rica...

.... single women indulging in sexual behaviour are frowned upon in Costa Rica. According to legislation, unattached women are legally forbidden from indulging in any form of and 'any type of lewd activities or behaviour' with a man.

... keeping a bawdy house is a crime in San José and those who break the law may be charged for *'keeping a place for the practice of indecency'*.

... an ancient law proclaimed that adulterers were beaten and then drowned.

In Ecuador...

... a young bride can be returned to her parents if her husband discovers she is not a virgin on their wedding night.

... a woman may legally dance in public wearing nothing more than a piece of gauze covering her belly button.

In Egypt...

... legislation stands that should any man in the town of Doha Qara surprise a naked woman while changing or bathing, then she must cover up her face rather than her body.

... 6,000 years ago rape was punishable with castration. A woman found guilty of adultery would find herself without a nose, the thinking being that without a nose it would be more difficult for her to find someone to share in her adulterous ways.

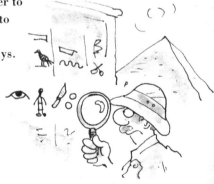

... and just as in Ecuador a law banned women from belly dancing unless their navel was covered with a piece of gauze.

In El Salvador...

... 'any married woman who lies with a man who is not her husband' can receive a fine and a six-year term in prison.

... in Santa Ana, having sex with a relative is a serious offence. The violators are either exiled or hanged.

In France...

... kissing on trains is illegal.

... one punishment for an adulterous wife in medieval France was to make her chase a chicken through town, naked.

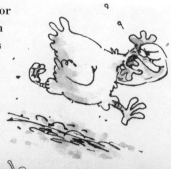

... provided that she was willing to join the opera, an 18th-century prostitute could be spared punishment.

In Great Britain...

... in Liverpool it is illegal for a woman to be topless in public unless she is employed as a clerk in a tropical fish store.

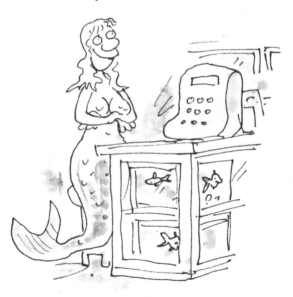

... according to an old law, having sex while riding a motorbike is banned in the City of London.

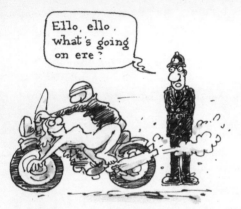

Ello, ello, what's going on ere?

... in the city of Birmingham ancient legislation states that it is illegal for any man and woman to have sex on the steps of any church after sunset – however there is no mention of it being prohibited before sunset.

... an ancient law dating back to 1288 stated that for each year known as a 'lepe yeare' any single lady could ask the man she liked to be her husband. Should he refuse without a good reason he would owe her a sum of money.

In Greece...

... adulterous men were once dealt with harshly. If caught in the act they had their pubic hair cut off and a large radish inserted into their rectum.

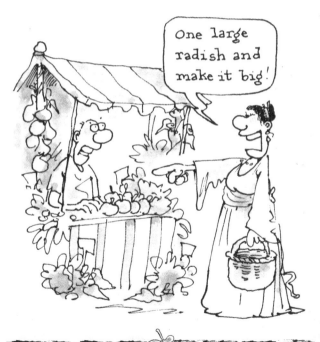

One large radish and make it big!

... in Athens, in the 6th century, legislator Solon passed a law which allowed fathers to sell their fornicating daughters into slavery.

In Guam...

... virgins once were not allowed to marry. Instead, fulltime fornicators were paid to travel around the country deflowering them.

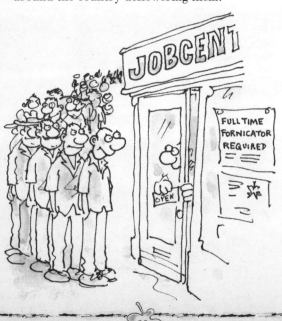

In Guatemala...

... single women accused of illicit lovemaking were once severely reprimanded. The law stated that whenever any female fornicators were seen in the streets they should be the stopped, spat upon and beaten up by the local citizens.

In Hong Kong...

... a betrayed wife is legally allowed to kill her adulterous husband but only by using her bare hands.

In India...

... long ago a fiancé was required to deflower his future bride if she died before the wedding. The girl could not be cremated until this ritual was carried out in front of the village priest.

... nude bathing is banned even in the holiday resort of Goa.

... because it is believed that carrot seeds have contraceptive qualities, women in the Indian state of Rajastan are encouraged to eat them.

In Iran...

... the law in Iran suggests that sex play between
men and wild animals is not recommended,
especially when it involves a lioness.

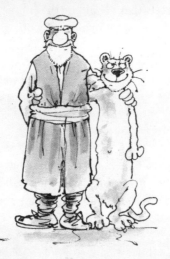

In Israel...

... no person is allowed to dress or undress in a
room with the light switched on.

... there is no legal way for any man named
Cohen to marry a divorced woman.

In Italy...

... in Naples a man is allowed to have as many mistresses as he wishes, provided that his wife knows, and that he can afford to maintain his wife and mistress in the lifestyle to which they are accustomed.

... men can be arrested for wearing skirts.

... in Osnago, northern Italy, legislators decided to sanction a law restricting how long couples were allowed to kiss one another in the local park. It seems that five seconds was long enough and anyone who went over that limit was committing a crime.

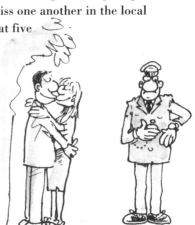

Loony Sex Laws

... in the 16th and 17th centuries the amount prostitutes could charge depended on how high their heels were. As a result a law was passed prohibiting women from wearing high heels.

... in medieval times the Romans knew how to deal with a rapist. For a first offence they would crush his testicles between two stones. For a second offence ... oh, yes, there was never any second offence!

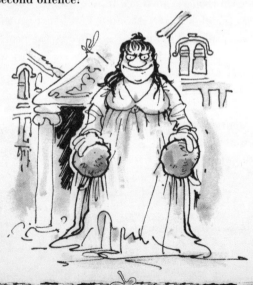

In Indonesia...

... decapitation is the penalty for anyone caught masturbating.

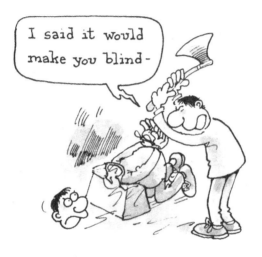

In Jordan...

... there is a curfew on the amount of sexual activity conducted between a man and his wife. Law designates that a man should make love to his wife at least once every four months.

In Laos...

... a law once was passed banning any Laos national inviting a fellow national of the opposite sex to one's hotel room.

In Lebanon...

... any Lebanese woman caught fornicating with a wild or domesticated animal must be executed.

In Mexico...

... a long time ago married couples in Durango could only have sex depending on the wife's menstrual cycle. A strict timetable was set out and sexual relations could only occur after 12 days into her cycle. This was so that five days had elapsed from the onset of the menstrual flow and seven days had elapsed for 'purification'. After the 12 days had elapsed, the woman had to bathe and only then could the couple recommence sex. However, the man was banned from touching his wife in any manner with his hands! The penalty for anyone violating this was death.

In the Middle East...

... marriage contracts in some places pledge that the wife is a virgin when she weds. Should this turn out not to be true then the husband is at liberty to have the marriage annulled.

... by law, if a husband is unable to make love to his wife, then she may have the marriage annulled and the husband in turn must pay her damages which are generally one half of the dowry as stated in the marriage contract.

... the consequence for any Muslim wife who refuses her husband sex is not be given any food to eat and any clothing other than what she is wearing. She must not ask her husband for sex at any time in the future and if he feels like it, the husband is at liberty to throw her out on the streets. Should the husband decide to divorce her, then by law, he must pay damages that represent part or all of her dowry.

In Nepal...

... lawmakers proclaimed it a crime to watch movies that displayed the pubic area of men and women or scenes of simulated lovemaking. Kissing on screen was also banned between actors from Nepal, Bangladesh and Macao!

In the Netherlands ...

... prostitution is legal, therefore anyone deriving income from it must declare it and pay tax on it.

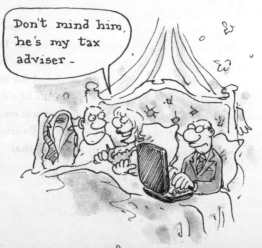

Don't mind him, he's my tax adviser –

In Nicaragua...

... divorce is the only option in Matagalpa for a man whose wife is guilty of adultery. However, should the wife catch her husband in bed with another woman, divorce is not even an option. The law states that such things are simply *expected to happen* when it comes to men.

In Panama...

... homosexuality is not tolerated. The law declares, '*If any of these males who commit this vile practice against nature with other males, he shall be degraded and shall remain in perpetual exile.*' The penalty meted out for homosexual behaviour is castration. The law also covers people who aren't homosexual themselves but who associate with homosexuals – guilt by association brings a penalty of a shaven head, 100 lashes and banishment.

In Paraguay...

... if a man catches his wife in bed with somebody else he is legally entitled to kill his wife and her lover, but only if he acts immediately.

In Peru...

... an archaic piece of legislation dating back to 1583, and passed by the third provisional council of Lima, reads: *'If there is anyone among you who commits sodomy, sinning with another man or with a boy or beast ... Let it be known that it carries the death penalty.'*

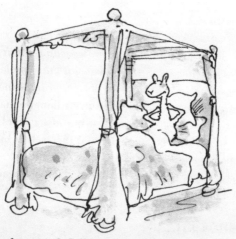

... the use of chilli sauce and similar hot spices added to prison food is outlawed. These items are thought to be aphrodisiacs and therefore unsuitable for pent-up inmates.

... sodomy has long been a serious offence. A person who has engaged in this act is dragged through the streets on a rope. Hanging comes next before the corpse is burned, fully clothed. This is said to symbolise the sodomite's total destruction.

... unmarried young men are prohibited from having a female alpaca live in their homes or apartments.

In Poland...

... in the city of Krakow having sex with animals is not regarded as a crime. However law dictates that those who do so three times are shot in the head.

In Puerto Rico...

... unmarried couples have no legal status but their offspring do and must be maintained by their unmarried parents until they are at least 21.

In Qatar...

... all forms of contraception are strictly forbidden because Qatar needs more males to work and more females to bear and raise children.

... if an unmarried woman becomes pregnant she is prohibited from using any hospital in the region, or from calling for any medical assistance. Her only options are either to do without health care or leave the country.

... in Doha, if a man surprises a naked Muslim woman while bathing or dressing she must first cover her face, not her body.

In Russia...

... the police were once allowed to 'beat peeping toms soundly'.

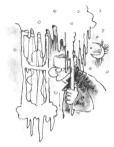

In Saudi Arabia...

...kissing in public is illegal.

... it is against the law for a woman to appear in public without a male relative or guardian present.

... the body is very sacred in the eyes of the Muslim religion and as such people are banned from looking at the genitals of a corpse. Likewise the same law applies to undertakers. Sex organs of the deceased must be covered with a piece of wood or a brick at all times.

... under no circumstances can any form of contraception be brought into the country. Anyone caught smuggling birth-control pills, condoms, or other contraceptive devices can expect to receive a six-month prison sentence.

... adulterers are punished by being tied into a cloth sack and then stoned to death, or alternatively the woman is shot in front of her lover, who is then publicly beheaded.

... male doctors may not examine women and female doctors cannot examine men.

In Singapore...

... pornography is illegal

... walking around your home naked is considered pornographic and so is unlawful.

... unless used as a form of foreplay, oral sex is forbidden.

In the Solomon Islands...

... should a Kurtatchi woman inadvertently expose her genitals, the law clearly states the following: *that it may be expected and will be understood if any man who is nearby at that moment in time sexually assaults her.*

Loony Sex Laws

In South Africa...

... repressive sex laws have been in existence for many years, largely as a result of apartheid to ensure racial purity. In 1965 the Chairman of The Censor Board had the film *Debbie* banned because he was under the impression that Afrikaner women did not become pregnant before marriage. When he was informed that this was not the case, the censorship was dropped.

... prostitution is illegal. However, this did not prevent up to 200 prostitutes once being allowed to work in the harbour area of Cape Town where they were registered with the authorities under the occupation of 'port hostesses'. Eventually this was banned as they were considered a fire and safety hazard on board ships carrying hazardous cargo (presumably because they enjoyed smoking after sex).

In Swaziland...

... in 1985 it was made illegal to have sex at Kadl-Padl hot springs, as the tourist hot spot had also become a popular place for couples to act out their sexual fantasies. The penalty was up to one year in jail.

In Sweden...

... whilst prostitution is legal in Sweden it is illegal for anyone to use the services of a *'lady of the night'*.

... it is legal for Swedes to go into photo booths and take topless photos. But full frontal photos are illegal.

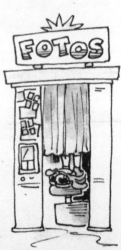

In Syria...

... a man is forbidden to look at the body of a woman who is not his wife and vice versa.

In Tasmania...

... according to an old law, when one's husband died they made sure he was never forgotten by his wife. To re-enforce this local officials authorised a law whereby widows were requested to wear their dead husband's penis around their neck for a period of time after his death.

In Thailand...

... free vasectomies have been available every year since 1981 in honour of the king's birthday.

.... it is illegal to leave your house if you are not wearing underwear.

In Tibet...

... many years ago Tibetan law required all women to prostitute themselves in order to gain sexual experience prior to marriage.

Loony Sex Laws

In the UAE...

... in Abu Dhabi, the police can arrest a person for 'committing an action that would be harmful to the general public'. Something as innocent as a man kissing a woman on her cheek in a public place would incur a penalty of ten days in jail for both parties.

In Uruguay...

... if a husband catches his wife in bed with another man then, according to the law, he has one of two options: he can either kill his wife and lover or slice off his wife's nose and castrate her lover.

... a husband isn't permitted to make love to his wife whilst she is menstruating, nor can he touch any part of her body between the waist and knees. If he does so he is both fined and publicly humiliated by receiving 200 lashes.

In the USA...

... did you know that:

In some states there are still laws which prohibit kissing.

Impotence is grounds for divorce in 24 states in the USA.

America has more laws governing sexual behaviour than every country in Europe combined.

In Alabama...

... in the township of Linden it was decreed that all women of uncertain chastity had to be off the streets by 9pm.

... an ancient law, sanctioned no doubt to protect the virginity of young girls, fixed a $300-500 fine and a six-month jail term for anyone who endeavoured to entice or employ a young girl aged between 10-18 years for immoral means.

... according to a 1950 anti-obscenity law, the exhibition of anyone naked or in a substantially naked state, except that of a babe in arms, was prohibited in the township of Irondale.

... a repealed law once strictly enforced in bygone days was that men were banned from spitting in front of a member of the opposite sex after 4pm in the evening.

... incestuous marriages are legal

... in the township of Anniston an old law bans women from using promises of a sexual nature in order to settle bets on games of pool. And they are also banned from initiating any sexual advances whilst hanging around a pool hall.

... don't even contemplate smuggling sex toys into Alabama, because they are banned.

... there is an ancient law banning men from trying to seduce *'a chaste woman by means of temptation, arts, deception, flattery or a promise of marriage'*.

In Arizona...

... in the township of Cottonwood lawmaker's sanctioned legislation against any couples found to be making love in cars with flat tyres. The penalties incurred read:

Should the car be parked and the couple were caught engaged in sexual activity in the front seats, then the penalty was a $25 fine.

Should the car be parked and the couple were caught engaged in sexual activity in the back seats, then the penalty was doubled to a $50 fine. However, should the couple be caught making love while driving the vehicle with flat tyres then the fine jumped to $100 for the first offence and $150 for any further offence thereafter.

... the law was once very strict regarding unmarried adults who had sex and if caught could spend the next three years in jail.

... all women were once banned from wearing corsets in the township of Nogales.

... men were once banned in Alexandria from making love to their wives if they had the odour of sardines, garlic or onion on their breath.

...in the eyes of the Arizona State Supreme Court female breasts were not considered as being private *parts* and so, in its worldly wisdom, it issued a law deeming that it was perfectly acceptable for women to go topless in public.

... women are banned from wearing suspenders in some of the smaller towns in Arizona.

In Arkansas...

... an old law dating back centuries banned flirting with opposite members of sex on the streets of Little Rock. Anyone caught could expect to spend at least 30 days in prison.

… acts of adultery were once regarded as criminal. The penalty for those who committed it was a fine ranging anywhere from $20 to $100.

… until 1994 it was not illegal for a man to molest a woman in public by fondling her breasts.

In California...

… legislation once required couples to wipe their lips with rose water before they were allowed to kiss.

… an old law stated that when two people were engaged in foreplay it was illegal for either partner to reach an orgasm before the other.

… cats and dogs have to be licensed before having sex.

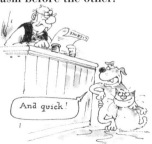

And quick!

... until 1975 it was decreed that husbands and wives could both expect a jail sentence of 15 years if they were found to be engaging in certain sexual practices. Oral sex, even in private, was expressly prohibited.

... in Beverly Hills, according to an old law, '*No male person shall make remarks to, or concerning, or cough or whistle at, or do any other act to attract the attention of any woman upon, or travelling along, any of the sidewalks.*'

... a man is legally entitled to strike his wife with a leather belt or strap in Los Angeles. However, the belt must be no wider than two inches across, unless he has his wife's consent to beat her with a wider strap.

... in San Francisco legislation was once passed banning people from using their underwear when cleaning their car.

… an edict once existed banning women from entering a gymnasium where men might be observed standing before mirrors.

In Colorado…

… lawmakers in Cattle Creek banned any husband or wife from making love while bathing 'in any river or stream'.

… in the township of Local, county legislators once banned men from kissing women when they were sleeping.

In Connecticut…

… a law once existed that stated it was a felony for a man to write love letters to an unmarried girl if her parents had previously disapproved of him.

… an odd law exists that makes absolutely no distinction between married and unmarried couples and forbids any 'private sexual behaviour between consenting adults'.

In Delaware...

... according to an old statute, getting married on a dare in the township of Lewes is grounds for annulment.

... legislation was passed requiring that every minor had to inform his or her parents before engaging in sexual intercourse.

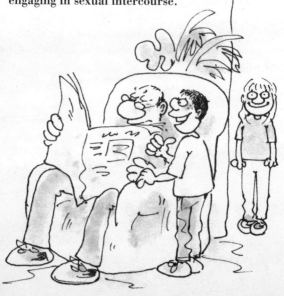

Loony Sex Laws

In Florida...

...walking or jogging topless within 150ft of the beach is illegal.

... it is illegal for women to expose more than two thirds of her bottom at the beach. If the bikini doesn't cover at least one third of her rear end a $500 fine can be imposed.

... stage nudity is banned in Sanford with the exception of 'bona fide' theatrical performances. Any persons violating this ordinance will be fined $100.

... an old statute once banned a man from kissing his wife's breasts.

... oral sex could get you a 20-year prison sentence.

... prostitution is dealt with by giving prostitutes spending money, a five-year banishment and a bus ticket out of town.

… an old statute states that one may not commit any 'unusual acts' with another person … there is no information as to what 'unusual acts' might mean.

… a bizarre law can be found on the statutes whereby it was considered an offence to shower naked!

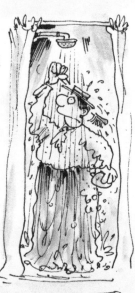

… exotic dancers in Tampa are banned from exposing their breasts whilst performing 'topless dancing'. Furthermore during their lap-dancing performances they must be at least 6ft away from a patron.

… it is a legal requirement in Satellite Beach that: *'Persons may not appear in public clothed in liquid latex.'*

... it is illegal for anyone to have sexual relations with a porcupine.

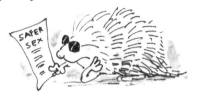

... if you're a single, divorced, or widowed woman, you are prohibited from parachute jumping on Sunday afternoons.

... a bygone law stated that: *'It is a crime for a man to be seen out and about in Florida with a 'visible' erection.'*

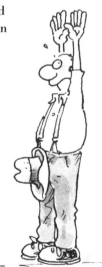

In Georgia...

... females in Columbus are not allowed to sit on their outdoor porch in an undignified manner.

... for owners of clothing stores in the city of Columbus the law decrees that whenever changing the clothes of a mannequin in a storefront the shades must be down.

... it is illegal for unmarried couples to have sexual intercourse.

... on a Sunday, erotic dancing is banned in the municipality of Roswell.

... sex toys are banned.

... it is illegal to be caught swimming in the nude anywhere in the vicinity of Georgetown. Offenders are transported to the outskirts of town and left to fend for themselves. And if they partake in any sexual activity whilst skinny dipping, they are covered with paint, attached to an ass and transported out of the town where they are left and told never to return.

In Hawaii...

... to be seen in public wearing only swimming
trunks and little else is an act of indecency.

In Idaho ...

... any police officer in Coeur d'Alene who
suspects that sex is taking place in a parked
vehicle must always drive up from behind, honk
his horn three times, and then wait two minutes
before getting out of his vehicle to investigate.

... legislators decided that engaging in a public
display of affection for any longer than 18
minutes was a crime.

In Illinois...

... protesting naked in front of the state city hall
is quite permissible on the proviso the person is
under the age of 17 and has a legal permit.

.... It is illegal in Minoola to remove one's clothes
and expose yourself during daylight or twilight
hours, even if simply for the purposes of taking a
bath.

Loony Sex Laws

... all bachelors should be called master, not mister, when addressed by women.

... it is against the law to make love on your wedding day while out fishing or hunting in Oblong.

In Indiana...

... anyone enticing, alluring, instigating or in any way helping a person under the age of 21 to masturbate was once considered a criminal offence.

... the law states that any male over the age of 18 years may be arrested for statutory rape if the passenger in his car is not wearing her socks and shoes and is under the age of 17.

... oral sex is banned.

In Iowa...

... kisses may last no more than five minutes.

.... a law prohibits men who dress up in female clothes from wearing shoes with heels more than two and a quarter inches high.

.... In the city of Ottumwa the law states is it unlawful for any male within the limits of the city to wink at any female person with whom he is unacquainted.

... kissing strangers in Cedar Rapids is a criminal act.

... husbands in the township of Ames should be aware that after making love to your wife, you are banned from taking more than three mouthfuls of beer whilst lying in bed or even when holding her in your arms.

In Kansas...

... according to an obscure 1901 city ordinance: *'The police can pick up any unattended females if they are "in the streets or any public place without lawful business and without giving a good accounting of themselves".'*

... should a man be caught patronising a prostitute he can expect a hefty fine of $500 and a one-month term in jail.

.... sex aids, such as vibrators, are illegal.

In Kentucky...

... certain townships have prohibited marrying the same man three times.

In Louisiana...

... couples shopping for a new bed are not permitted to adopt the 'try before you buy' test. According to the wording of the edict legislators describe the test as *'making love on it, or even simulating this activity'*.

... streaking with the intent of arousing the desires of minors carries a sentence of up to five years in the state penitentiary plus a $2,000 fine. Streaking with the intent solely of arousing sexual desire brings the violator a $100 fine and one year in prison. Should the streaker prove beyond any doubt to the court that he or she had no 'lascivious intent' then no fine or jail sentence is imposed.

In Maine...

... a taxi driver cannot charge a passenger who, in return for a ride home from a nightclub or other establishment serving alcoholic beverages, provides him with sexual favours.

In Maryland...

... condoms cannot be purchased from vending machines unless they are dispensed in places where alcoholic beverages are sold for consumption on the premises.

... in Halethorpe kissing for more than one second is illegal. (Who's timing them?)

... oral sex is banned.

In Massachusetts...

... a law once banned women from assuming the superior position in sexual intercourse.

... according to an ancient law married couples in Salem are banned from sleeping naked in rented rooms.

In Michigan...

... a law passed in Detroit in the early part of the 20th century stated that, *'any sexual relationships taking place between couples are not allowed to take place in an automobile unless the act takes place while the vehicle is parked on the couple's own property.'*

... male drivers in Detroit are banned from 'ogling' women whilst their car is in motion.

... an old statute which exists in Sturgis actually bans *large females* (no definition of 'large' is given) who are seeking to marry from using 'handbills' as a means of advertising for a spouse.

... for any acts of adultery records propose a fine of as much as $5,000 and that doesn't include a possible prison sentence of five years.

... irrespective of whether a married couple were happy living together or not, an old law was enforced in which it was clearly written that they either *'live together or face imprisonment'*

... forget about serenading your girlfriend in Kalamazoo ... it is illegal.

... adultery is illegal but punishment can only be inflicted if the affected partner proposes the complaint. And furthermore, if the offence was committed over a year before the actual complaint was made, no prosecution may take place.

... should a man attempt to corrupt and seduce an unmarried girl, the law states that he can risk spending up to five years in prison.

In Minnesota...

... underwear from both sexes could not be hung out to dry on the same clothesline.

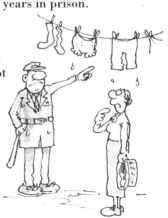

Loony Sex Laws

... oral sex is banned.

... it is not permitted in Alexandria for a husband to make love to his wife if he has the smell of onions, sardines or garlic on his breath. And should his wife demand that he brush his teeth then legally he must do so!

... sleeping naked is illegal.

... it is illegal for men to have any intimate sexual relations with a live fish.

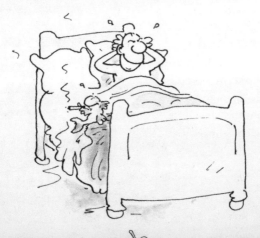

... in the township of Minnetonka, if a person persuaded another to enter a massage therapy business after the hour of 11pm, it was considered a criminal act.

... in the legal archives of St Paul, an ancient piece of legislation states that: '*no person shall appear in a public place or street in a state of nudity, nor in a dress not belonging to his or her sex, nor in any indecent or lewd dress, nor make any indecent exposure of his or her person, nor commit any obscene or filthy act, nor commit any lewd indecent, immoral or insulting conduct, behaviour, nor utter any lewd, indecent immoral or insulting language.*'

In Mississippi...

... a man is not allowed to seduce a woman by promising to marry her.

... state officials ordained that there is a fine of $500 and/or a six-month term in jail should a couple reside together under the same roof whilst not married or have sexual relations with someone that is not their spouse.

... an old edict stipulates that it is against the law for a man to be sexually aroused in public.

... an old law states that: *'if riding in a vehicle with a member of the opposite sex and both are bare footed then in the eyes of the law you are legally married.'*

In Missouri...

... anal intercourse is banned in Bexley.

... cross-dressing in Ironton is illegal.

... it is illegal in Oxford for a woman to strip off her clothing while standing in the front of a man's picture.

... women are prohibited from wearing corsets in Merryville because, 'the privilege of admiring the curvaceous, unencumbered body of a young women should not be denied to the normal, red-blooded American male'.

In Montana...

… sexual activity is banned between members of the opposite sex in the front garden of any home in Bozeman after dusk … but only if the lovemakers are nude!

… a woman cannot dance on a table in a saloon or bar unless she has on at least three pounds and two ounces of clothing – so who was weighing?

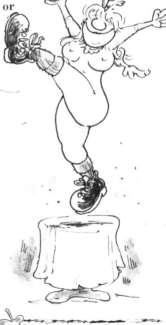

In Nebraska...

... the owner of every hotel in this state is required to provide each guest with a clean and pressed nightshirt. No couple, even if they are married, may sleep together in the nude or have sex unless wearing one of these clean, cotton nightshirts.

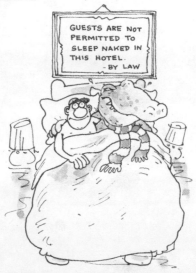

GUESTS ARE NOT PERMITTED TO SLEEP NAKED IN THIS HOTEL.
- BY LAW

... the act of buggery can result in a minimum of a 20-year prison sentence.

In Nevada...

... any member of
the Nevada Legislature
who conducts business
wearing a penis
costume while
it is in session
is violating
the law.

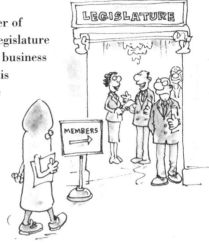

... city fathers in the township of Eureka banned
any man with a moustache from kissing a
woman.

... it is illegal to have a 'house of ill fame' within
400 yards of a church or school.

.... having casual sex without a condom is illegal.
Safe sex is imperative as there are over 35 legal
bordellos, not to mention the illegal ones. As a

result legislation was passed ordering each brothel to have a supply of condoms readily available and it is compulsory that they are used within these establishments.

In New Hampshire...

... lesbian sex is not adulterous when cited in a divorce action because the Supreme Court has ruled that the definition of adultery requires sexual intercourse.

In New Jersey...

... courting couples in Liberty Corner must refrain from sexual intercourse in parked cars as they can face jail terms, especially if the car horn is inadvertently sounded during the act.

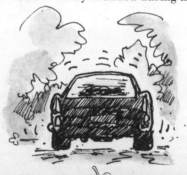

In New Mexico...

... it is permissible for couples in Carlsbad to have sex in public during their lunch break, so long as they are in a parked car with curtains drawn.

... state officials once ordered the removal of over 400 words to be cut from *Romeo and Juliet*, as they considered them to be of a sexually explicit nature.

In New York...

... at one time, any man caught turning around on a city street and flirting with a woman was fined $25. Should the same man be convicted twice of the same crime then he would be forced to wear a 'pair of horse-blinders' wherever and whenever he went outside for a stroll.

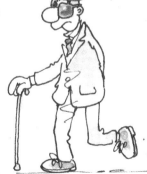

... women may go topless in public unless it is for 'business' purposes.

... an old ordinance stipulates that women should not be seen wearing 'body hugging clothing'.

... it is illegal to have consensual sodomy with anyone unless you are married to him or her.

In North Carolina...

... it is illegal for a man to peep through a window at a woman, but it is not against the law for a woman to peep into a room occupied by a man – nor is it a violation if a man peeps at another man.

... extra-marital sex is illegal.

... massage parlours are banned in Hornytown.

... if an unmarried man and woman go to a hotel or motel and register themselves as 'Mr and Mrs' then according to state law they are legally husband and wife.

... all couples staying overnight in a hotel must have a room with double beds with a distance of at least 2ft between them. Making love in the space between the beds is not allowed.

... having sex in a graveyard is an offence.

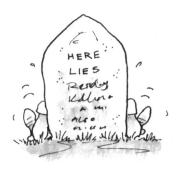

Loony Sex Laws

In Ohio...

... anal intercourse is banned in Cincinnati.

... an old statute found in the township of Oxford prohibits women from stripping off clothing whilst standing in front of a man's picture.

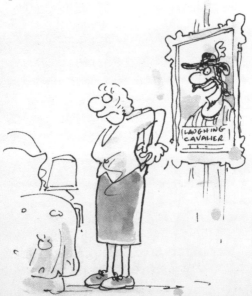

... male skating instructors are banned from having sexual relationships with their female students. This edict only applies to male teachers.

... a law was passed banning women from wearing patent leather shoes in Cleveland in case a man might catch a glimpse of something he shouldn't.

In Oklahoma...

... oral sex is a misdemeanour and punishable with a one-year jail term and a $2,500 fine.

... if anyone is arrested for soliciting a prostitute then he will have his or her name and picture shown on TV.

... it was once considered statutory rape for a man over the age of 18 to have sex with a woman under the age of 18 ... provided she was a virgin. If she was not a virgin, then rape had not taken place, unless the said was under 16. If both parties were under 18, then the law did not apply!

... it was once illegal to have sex before you were married.

... women are banned in Schulter from gambling in the nude, while wearing lingerie, or if covered only in a towel.

... in the township of Clinton it was illegal to masturbate whilst watching two people having sex in a car. The peeping tom could expect a fine and a term in jail for *'molesting a vehicle'*.

In Oregon...
... in Willowdale men can be fined for using profane language during intercourse with their wives. Their wives can say what they like.

... in Salem it is illegal for patrons of establishments that feature nude dancing to be within 2ft of the dancers.

In Pennsylvania...

… a special law was passed governing sexual activities in toll collection booths on the Pennsylvania Turnpike. The law, which pertained only to female toll collectors, banned them from engaging in sex with a truck driver in the confines of a booth. Any woman violating this law would be fired for *'behaviour unbecoming an employee'*. If for any reason the transgressor was later reinstated, she was not allowed back pay.

… it is illegal for over 16 women to live in a house together since this is thought to constitute a brothel. Yet up to 120 men can live together without breaking the law.

… men living in Allentown are not allowed to become sexually aroused in public.

In Rhode Island...

… legislators in the 1970s proposed there would be a $2 tax imposed on every act of sexual intercourse.

In South Carolina...

... an old law ordained that if a man promised to marry someone, then he was legally bound to do so.

In South Dakota...

... prostitutes were once banned from plying their trade in a covered wagon.

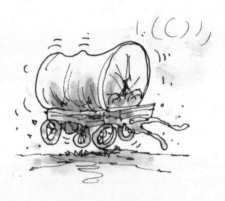

... all hotel rooms in Sioux Falls must have twin beds only. If a room is booked by a couple on a one-night-only basis, then the beds must be at least 2ft apart. It is also illegal to make love on the floor between the beds.

… anal sex is punishable by a $500 fine and a five-year prison term.

In Tennessee...

… women in Dyersburg are not allowed to call a man for a date.

… the law in Skullbone bans a woman from pleasuring a man while he is sitting behind the wheel of any moving vehicle. Should a man be stopped and found with the front of his pants undone he can be fined a minimum of $50 and serve 30 days in jail.

… it is illegal for a man in Nashville to be sexually aroused in public.

In Texas...

… flirting is banned in San Antonio.

… homosexual oral sex and/or sodomy is banned in Kingsville. It is legal between heterosexuals.

... unmarried adults who are apprehended while having sex are charged with a misdemeanour and given a $500 fine.

... 16-year-old divorced girls are prohibited from talking about sex during high school extracurricular activities.

... no one other than a *'registered pharmacist'* may sell condoms or other kinds of contraceptive *'upon the streets or other places'*. Anyone who does will be prosecuted for the 'unlawfully practising medicine'.

... it is illegal to possess realistic dildos, vibrators and artificial vaginas. If someone is in possession of seven or more of these than they can be charged as it as considered a class A crime.

In Utah...

... within the boundaries of Tremonton no woman may have sex with a man while riding in an ambulance. This is considered a sexual misdemeanour and her name may be published in the local newspaper. The male is apparently considered faultless.

... sexual intercourse between consenting but unmarried adults is regarded as a class B misdemeanour and punishable by a $1,000 fine and six months in jail.

... daylight must be visible between dancing couples in Monroe.

... it is illegal for first cousins to marry before they reach the age of 65.

... state legislation outlaws all sex with anyone but your spouse. Next to adultery, oral and anal sex and even masturbation can lead to imprisonment. Polygamy, provided only the missionary position is used, is only a misdemeanour.

In Vermont...

... it is illegal in Beanville to publish, sell or give away a road map if it contains advertising of a *'lewd or lascivious nature'*. The ban specifically includes adverts for massage parlours and hot tubs, as both are believed to be of a *'sensual bent'*.

In Virginia...

... no one may have sex while riding in the sidecar of a motorcycle in Norfolk where an old ordinance bans it. Such activity is considered to be a *'licentious sexual act'*.

... a man can be sent to prison for one to ten years if he should cause his wife to become a prostitute.

... a law in the locality of Rombach states that all lights should be turned off when couples are engaging in sex.

... a man in Norfolk can face 60 days in jail for patting a woman's bottom.

... single men are not allowed to have sexual relations – so how do they learn?

... oral and anal sex is banned.

... in Norfolk there used to be a men-only job in the civil service for a corset inspector, because it was illegal for women to go out without wearing a corset.

In Washington...

... there is a law against having sex with a virgin under any circumstances (and that includes the wedding night!).

... sex with an animal is perfectly legal for men provided the animal does not exceed 40lbs in weight.

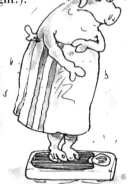

... the only acceptable sexual position in Washington DC is the missionary position. Any other sexual position is considered illegal.

... women who sit on mens' laps on buses or trains without placing a pillow between them face an automatic six-month jail term.

... men who deflower virgins in Auburn, regardless of age or marital status, may face up to five years in jail.

In Wisconsin...

... it is illegal for a man in Connersville to fire a gun when his female partner reaches orgasm.

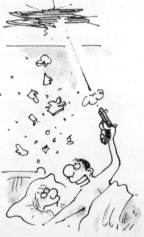

In Wyoming...

... couples in Newcastle are banned from having sex inside walk-in meat freezers.

... there are laws against anyone enticing, alluring, instigating or helping a person under 21 to masturbate. This activity is known in legal circles as an act of 'self pollution'.

In Venezuela...

... adultery is not necessarily a crime in Caracas. The length of time the couple have been married is a deciding factor. Providing the couple have been married for less than one year they can 'play around' and not be prosecuted. However after one year of marriage extra-marital sex is considered adulterous.

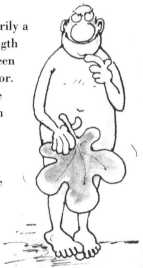

Loony Sex Laws

In Yemen ...

... adultery carries a sentence of public beheading.

... menstruation is important to a Muslim woman and so if she should bleed when having sex the man must instantly withdraw. Should he fail to do so an ancient law states he must make a financial contribution to the poor. If he himself is poor then he must proffer something, however little, to a beggar on the streets. But if he is a beggar himself the final and last resort is for him to beg God's forgiveness.